Anti-Aging White Beauty Secrets

Quick Guide to Looking 10 Years Younger

by Dr. Bola "LaLae" Show, M.D., M.B.A

the SOCIAL DIVA DOCTOR

LA LA SINCERELY™

Atlanta

First printing

This publication contains the opinions and ideas of its author. The author intends to offer information of a general nature. Any reliance on the information herein is at the reader's own discretion. No medical claims are made. Consult with your physician first if you have any medical condition and before starting any physical activity, nutritional, or other recommendations.

Any recommendations are made without any guarantee on the part of the author or the publisher.

LA LA SINCERELY INC. has allowed this work to remain exactly as the author intended, verbatim, without editorial input.

Hardcover 978-0-615-45470-2

PUBLISHED BY LA LA SINCERELY INC.
www.socialdivadoctor.com

LA LA SINCERELY

Atlanta
Printed in the United States of America

DEDICATION

By now, I'm enjoying my new found love of writing considering this is my second book. I don't take this for granted at all, but I give all the thanks to my God Almighty.

I hope you guys were motivated and inspired by my first book, *A Winner's Guide to Wearing These Many Hats: A Handbook to Making All Your Dreams & Passions Work For You.* If you haven't picked it up yet, please do so. You'll learn how to make every role you play in your life work for you while you follow your many dreams and passions. Your continuous support is always appreciated. Thank you!

ACKNOWLEDGMENTS

I am a big believer of being there for those who've been there for me from day one. With that being said and considering this is my second book, I would like to thank my team for being there with me from book number one to book number two. I have truly enjoyed working with you all.

Thanks to the models for being professional and looking gorgeous. To my Creative Director, you're amazing for continuing to capture my vision like no other and your creativity knocks the socks off my feet. Thanks for believing in fabulous possibilities.

CONTENTS

Introduction

It's with great excitement that I share with you my beauty secrets to looking 10 years younger. I've been asked by many to tell them what my beauty secrets are. People have wondered especially when I was in medical school how I managed to look 'stress-free' despite all the long hours of studying and examinations. Well, my answers have always been "I thank God," or "it's God." With those responses being true, I also bring it to their attention that it's the way I look at life. I don't associate myself with negativity or negative people. I try to be positive. Most importantly, I try to enjoy my life and be happy the best possible way I can. I think all that alone bring lots of happiness and youthfulness into your inner being, soul, mind, and skin. Your overall behavior and character traits can translate onto how your skin appears or its presentation. So if you're a miserable and angry person, and you spend most of your day being so, you will have a miserable and angry look for the most time. Your skin will take the beat from all the emotions involved.

I wrote this book to share with you that you don't have to spend a fortune to commit to daily beauty regime or to achieve youthful appearance. All you need is zero to few dollars. The best part is that you may already have some of the recommended beauty items in your cabinet. The goal here is to look amazing and 10 years younger without breaking the bank. I'm not a professional skin expert or dermatologist, but I have the medical knowledge, youthful skin, amazing beauty tips and secrets which I call the 'beauty cheat sheet' to looking 10 years younger.

In this book, you'll also learn my secret keywords to anti-aging. Some of the words are 'white,' 'hydrate,' and 'glossy.' These three words describe the importance and secret to looking 10 years younger. If you're not able to do all three, you'll find it hard to achieve your goal. At the same time, if you're able to apply all three in your daily beauty regimen, it will be difficult for your skin to easily go through the process of aging.

Introduction

I may have been gifted with amazing genes and youthful skin; I give the thanks to my heritage and mom who only looks a fraction of her age. You may not necessarily have good genes in your family, but you can achieve it now. It's never too late. I'll do my best to help you achieve amazing results with affordable price tags.

When I decided to write this book, I wanted to write something that wasn't out there on the book shelves or products that are readily used by many. As with everything I write about, I try to solve a problem instead of readdressing a problem. So I came up with unique, unusual, and affordable ways to looking 10 years younger by keeping everything white.

You may ask why white? It's a pretty simple concept, but it's a beauty secret at the same time. Let's think about it a little further. Assume you're now 45 years old. When you were 17 years old, weren't your eyes, teeth, and nails much whiter? Wasn't your hair sleeker, shinier, and healthier? Wasn't your skin much smoother, supple, hydrated, and radiant? I'm sure you'd quickly answer yes to all of these questions. But the problem and difference from when you were 17 and now 45 years old is because you've aged more. Not to make you sound older, but it's the truth. Unfortunately, we can't go back to how we looked when we were all teenagers, but we can still get close to achieving youthful appearances again. So this is where I'd like to help you achieve youthful appearance by implementing what I call my *white* anti-aging system to your daily beauty regimen.

My *white* anti-aging beauty system is for everyone. It's for all ages, skin types and for males and females who simply want to look their best. Beyond the *white* anti-aging secret, I'm also providing you with additional beauty regime which you can adopt in the comfort of your own home. It will literally take 10 years off your current age if you follow my recommendations. I know you'll find these beauty secrets to be effective and life changing while you're only one step away from discovering your youthful self.

Chapter 1

Whiter Teeth

Background: We all know a great set of teeth is an attractive thing; so you can imagine a mouth with missing, decayed, gingivitis, or discolored teeth. Absolutely, none of those are attractive or would be a choice you would prefer. There's something in particular about discolored teeth that equates aging.

Some personal behaviors can cost you a mouthful of white teeth. Many people have smoked cigarettes, chewed tobacco, drank coffee or red wine for many years. These behaviors can definitely result in discoloration of your teeth. This is where you'll have to start reversing the damage so you can still achieve whiter teeth. Follow my beauty steps below, and you'll be one step closer to your bright, beautiful teeth and smile.

Beauty Secrets:
1. **Basics: You simply want to achieve whiter teeth by doing what you normally do before which is to brush your teeth every day. Not everyone does this, but you need to <u>brush twice daily</u> in the morning and evening right before getting under the sheets. Doing so twice daily helps to minimize gingivitis and maintains long-lasting whiter teeth.**
2. **The key secret here is to use a <u>whitening system</u> that will help to not only clean your teeth each time you use it, but it will also help you to keep them 2-3 shades whiter. I recommend the Super Smile whitening system. It doesn't make your teeth sensitive as most do,**

and it doesn't have a nasty taste. The more you use it, the better results you'll achieve.

3. Another secret is to try <u>baking soda</u> to brighten your teeth. It's affordable and probably in your refrigerator right now.

4. Remember, be persistent, smile more, and you'll be amazed to see how this little change could make you look 10 years younger.

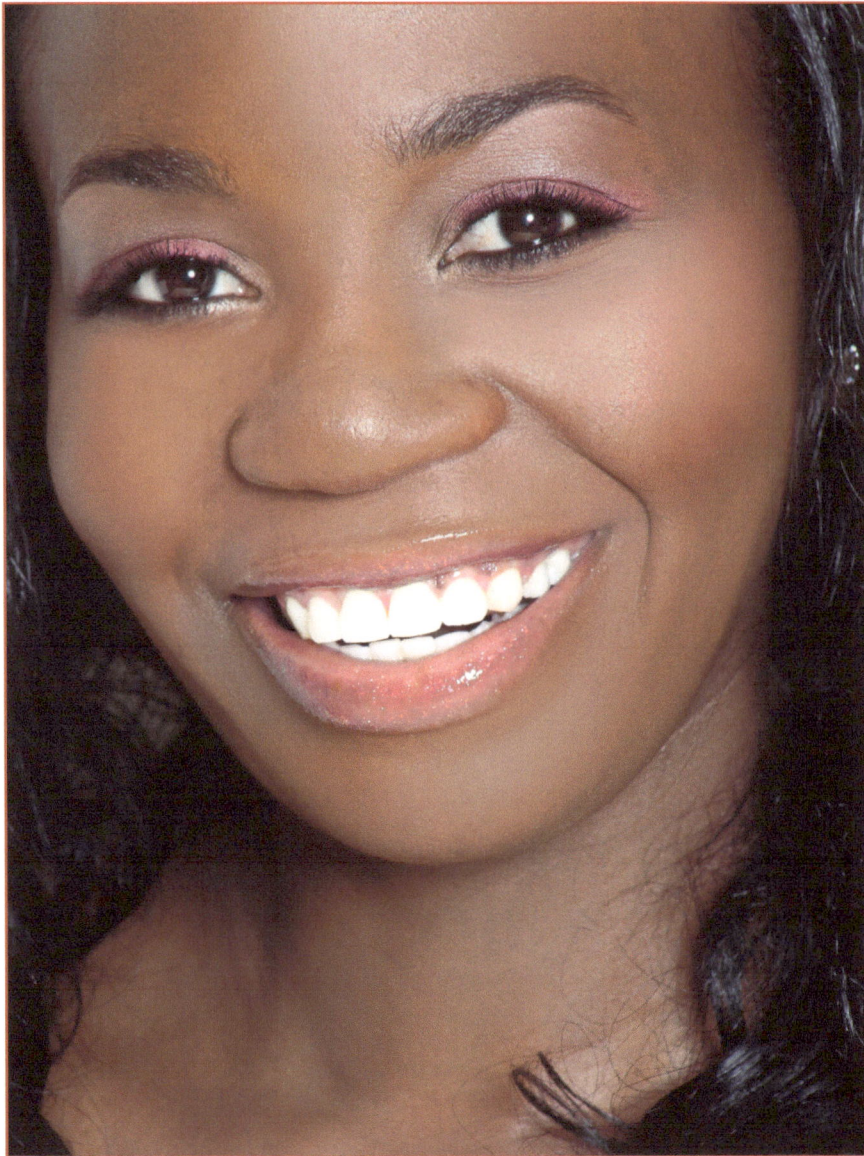

Chapter 2

Whiter Eyes

Background: Many don't necessarily associate youth with whiter eyes. What people don't know is that when their eyes are discolored, they look older and stressed out. No matter how much makeup you put on your face, a discolored pair of eyes is not attractive. This is the first thing that most people see when they meet you and they're talking to you and looking straight into your eyes. This can be intimidating knowing that you've aged eyes. It can also be costly to get a laser procedure to achieve whiter eyes, but in this book, we're talking all about looking younger without paying a lot.

Beauty Secrets:

1. **Basics: You need to avoid factors that can contribute to stressed-out eyes like too much alcohol, lack of sleep, stress, substance abuse drugs, and high blood pressure. These factors can either make your eyes red with ruptured veins, puffy with hyperpigmentation, or with yellowish discoloration. You simply want to <u>reduce alcohol</u> intake, get <u>more sleep</u> by going to bed early and finding what sleep schedule works best for you. You definitely should choose a <u>drug-free</u> life style, and <u>consult with your physician</u> to assess your blood pressure if you have symptoms like red eyes, blurry vision, nausea and vomiting, and headaches.**

2. The key secret to achieving whiter eyes instantly is to use an affordable '<u>Clear Eyes</u>' eye drops. Clear Eyes takes the redness out instantly, and you can get them for only $1-$2. 1-2 drops in each eye is all you need to achieve your instant whiter eyes. You may do this twice daily. Consult with your physician before doing this if you already have an underlying eye problem or medical problem which affects the eyes or ocular system.

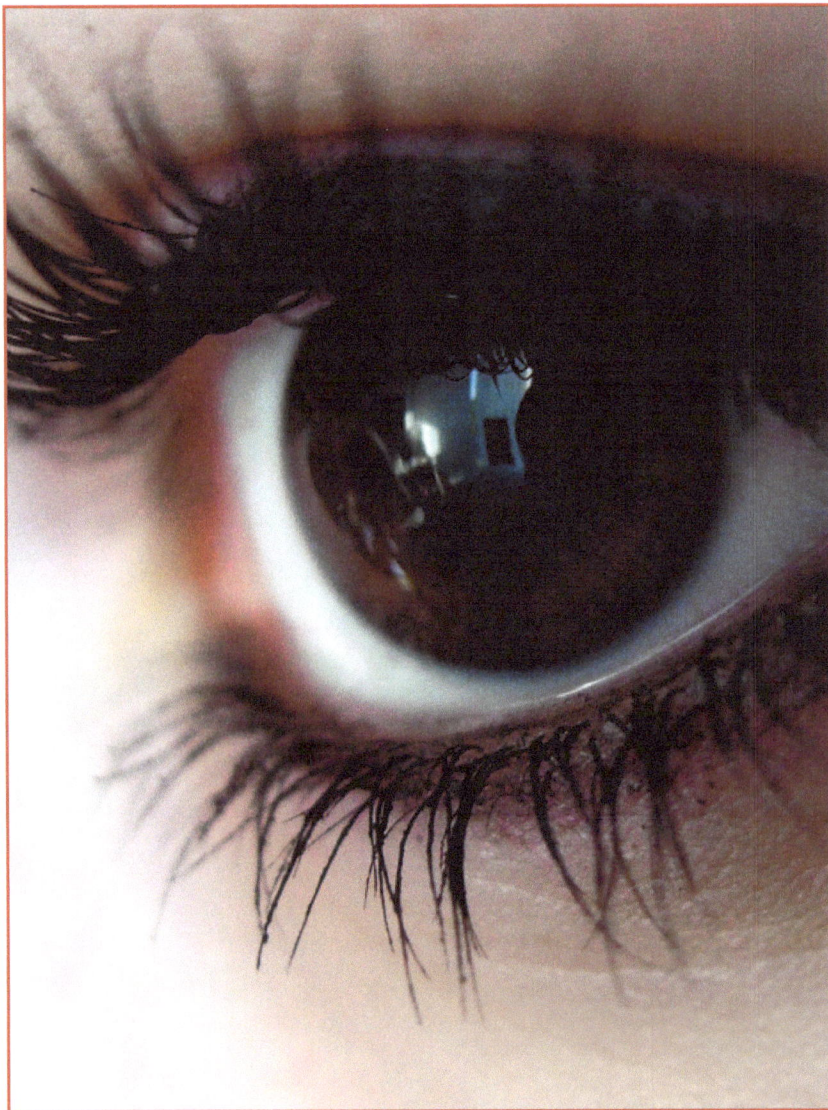

Chapter 3

Whiter Nails

Background: Achieving whiter nails goes along with whiter eyes. You may not realize it, but when you meet people, like with your eyes, you communicate with your hands. Hand gestures are behaviors of many either because they are nervous when speaking or simply because they just love to talk with their hands and are expressive.

A healthy set of hands are moistened and the nails are well groomed. If you want to look 10 years younger, keep your finger nails healthy and think "white." Our nails are usually tan in color. That's fine, but the idea behind it is that you want to keep it that color as often as you can. When you wear dark colors over your nails all the time, they make your nails appear aged. I'm not saying don't wear the reds, blacks, blues-- nail colors, I'm just saying lean towards the softer and whiter colors since they tend to give you a more youthful appearance. Colors like the whites or nudes, pinks, and any color in its lightest shade are most preferable to looking 10 years younger.

Beauty Secrets:
1. **Basics: Keep your <u>nails filed and nicely groomed</u> at all times. Keep a <u>nail filer</u> in your hand bag to quick-fix any emergency nail chips.**
2. **The key secret is to use <u>hair or body oils</u> as your hand lotion. They help to replenish your natural oils, and they instantly strengthen your troubled nails. If for any reason you're not able to use oils, use**

what you have like body lotions, but they must be very hydrating. The overall goal is to keep everything <u>hydrated</u>. You'll learn more about this in a later chapter.

3. Another secret as mentioned earlier is to think whiter nail colors. Besides using lighter nail colors for nail polish, I recommend using '<u>French</u>' nail tips occasionally or just French nail color. You don't have to go to the nail salon every two weeks. You can get the <u>opaque white</u> nail color, and apply it to your nails and use the clear color over it to keep it glossy and protected. This is what you call instant youth on your nails. If you want to see it for yourself, watch one of those jewelry shows on TV. Their hands are worth thousands of dollars. They can sell ANY jewelry on their fingers, and guess what nail colors they use?—nudes, clears, pinks, and French's. Why? It's youthful, attractive, and HOT!

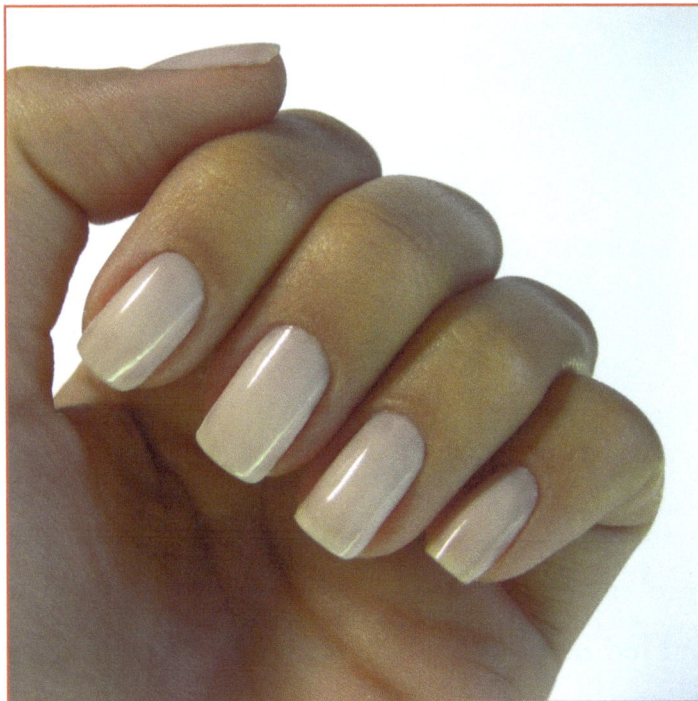

Chapter 4

All About the Hair

Background: Your hair can be an aging factor. Think about it—when you were a baby, your hair was probably super soft, healthy, and shiny. There's a reason why we look at babies and think they're the most beautiful creatures. Well, they are. It's not just because of their innocence and how wonderful they are. It's also about the features they have that we used to have, and we only wish we can get them all over again. Their hair, eyelashes, smile, skin, and more are all that we long for.

Wait no longer. You can achieve the youthful look by simply moisturizing and straightening your hair, trimming the ends, and coloring in darker shades. This time, the "white" rule changes. The darker your hair color is, the younger you appear. It's not that grey hair is bad. If the grey hair is monochromatic, then it's sexy too. But, let's face it. Not many of us want grey hair. I personally found that when I keep my perm and hair color fresh every month, it's amazing how much younger I look. It's the fresh look, the glisten and high-shine, the trim, and the freshly-crisped color that makes your hair a home-run. This shouldn't be expensive. You can buy a perm-relaxer box and dark color-rinse from your neighborhood drug store and do it yourself if you've always done it before, or if you have a hair dresser in your family, they can help you with it. If not, you can go to a hair school where you can get it done by students who are supervised at an affordable price.

Beauty Secrets:

1. **Basics:** Get your hair <u>shampooed, conditioned, trimmed, cut</u> frequently and as needed.

2. The key secret is to think of <u>high-shine, dark, straightened, sleek</u> hair. This is attainable by getting your <u>perm regularly</u> especially for coarse hair. The goal is to make sure your hair always looks like it's freshly done and trimmed. If you're able to do this as frequent as on a <u>monthly</u> basis, you'll be able to achieve instant youthful appearance and looking 10 years younger.

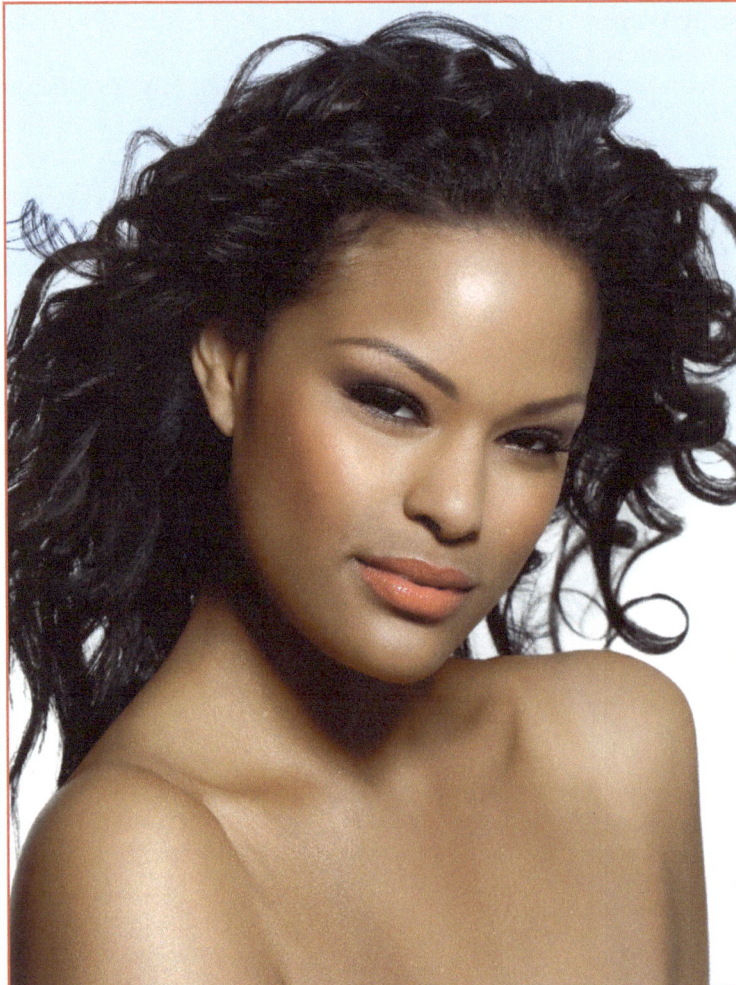

Chapter 5

The Trick Behind Ice Cubes

Background: This is another beauty secret of mine that isn't your regular cookie-cutter beauty regimen. It's not a huge discovery, but not many people know it works or to use it. You see, when you're tired, stressed, or old, your skin wrinkles. If you're a chronic smoker also, you're not left out. Your skin wrinkles a lot more. My secret is after washing your face with your regular beauty regimen, you want to blot dry with a clean facial towel. Then you apply ice cubes in a circular fashion. It helps to plump up your skin. The coldness is the trick as it closes the pores. Think about the scenario why you're being asked to wash your face with warm water and then with cold water before drying it. Or what about after getting a perm or a color-rinse, and warm water is used? Cold water is usually used thereafter to 'close' the hair follicles. The same logic when it applies to the face. You want to close the facial pores to prevent dirt from settling in, to prevent your beauty products from sinking into your skin, and to achieve a youthful look.

Beauty Secrets:
1. **Basics: <u>Wash your face twice daily</u> with a simple and mild cleansing system. Implementing a <u>facial scrub</u> every other day is fine. Avoid anything too abrasive or drying. You want moisture not drying effect.**

2. **The key secret is to apply <u>1-2 ice cubes</u> over a clean face by gently moving in a circular fashion twice daily. Apply from hairline to declitae. This helps to achieve a face and neckline with <u>pores that appear to have disappeared</u>. Your face will appear <u>supple and plump</u> like a baby's rear. It's like Botox for your face without the pain and cost. What you'll get is an instant youthful, soft, and radiant skin.**

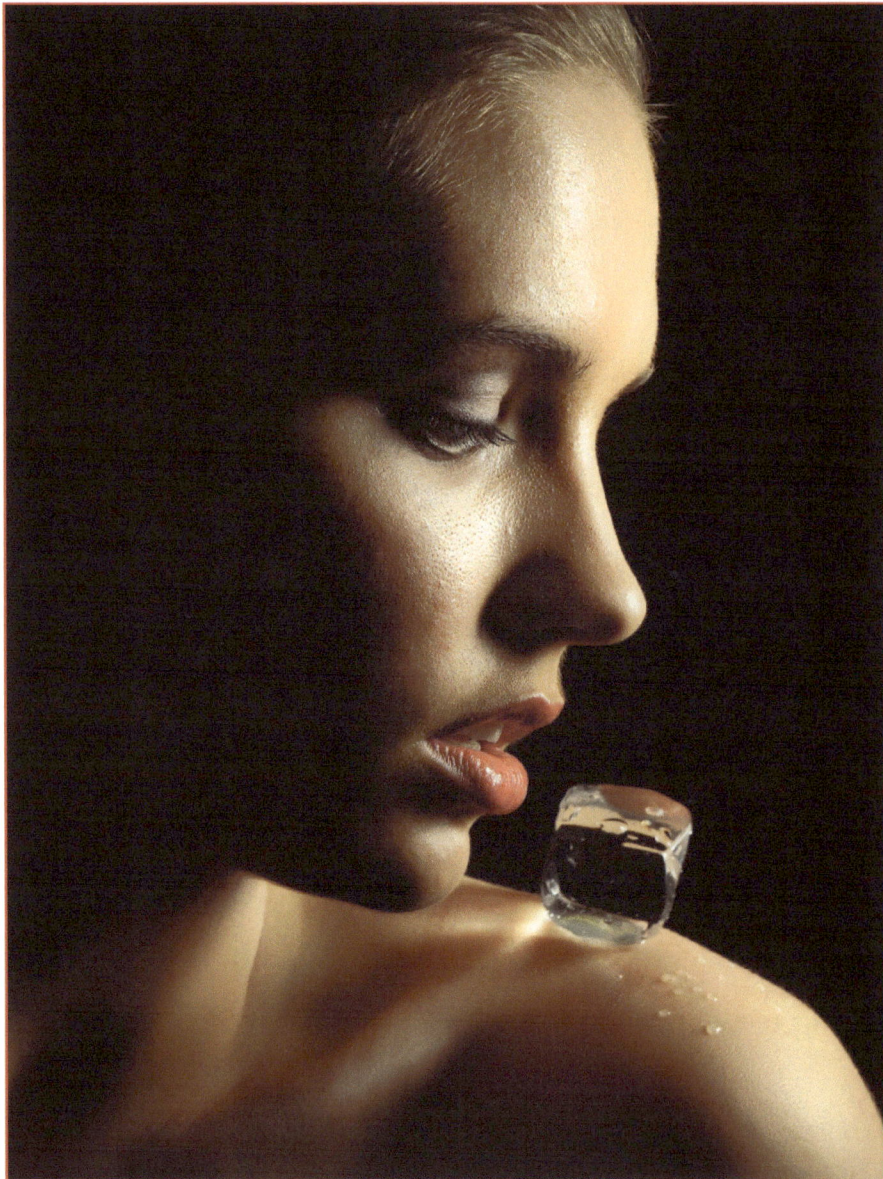

Chapter 6

Hydrate! Hydrate!! Hydrate!!!

Background: This chapter is placed somewhere in the middle of this book, but it's the most important chapter. What's important here is that you have to learn that hydration is the key to anti-aging. I'm sure you've heard the saying "dry skin equals aging skin." This is true, and this means because you've allowed your skin to be dry and scaly, it's started to look like you've aged and added 10 years to your age. The solution is to keep it moisturized and hydrated. Hydration means putting back water or moisture into the skin. You could imagine if you didn't have water to drink at all. The same applies to the skin. You want to take your skin seriously, and if you want to look younger, you will need to hydrate as much as you can. You can do so by either using moisturizer or serum. Serums are more potent than moisturizer, so they should be used closest to your skin, and then you can apply your moisturizer.

Beauty Secrets:

1.   **Basics: Take your baths and wash your face with mild and gentle cleanser. Avoid any alcohol ingredients. They would dry your skin and achieve the opposite of your goal.**

2.   **The key secret here is that you want to keep your face and body hydrated and not necessarily oily at all times. If you usually have dry skin, you can achieve hydration by buying an affordable, non-sensitive facial**

lotion from your local drug store. If you can afford it, buy a Dr Denese <u>anti-aging, hydrating facial serum</u>. If you can't afford either one, then I recommend to simply moisturize using good, old <u>Vaseline</u>. Remember, the key is to hydrate, and in this case, lubrication works. Don't forget to target the <u>upper and lower eye area</u>. This is where the aging shows the most.

3.   The same thing goes for your body. When your body is dry, your skin would appear scaly and old. You always want to have it moisturized by using a good <u>moisturizer with Aloe Vera, Vitamin E, or Shea Butter</u>. Either one of them is affordable, but if price is still a factor, again, go back to the good, old Vaseline. A tint of <u>olive oil</u> well blended to either the lotion or the Vaseline, creates great synergy for a fabulous moisturizer.

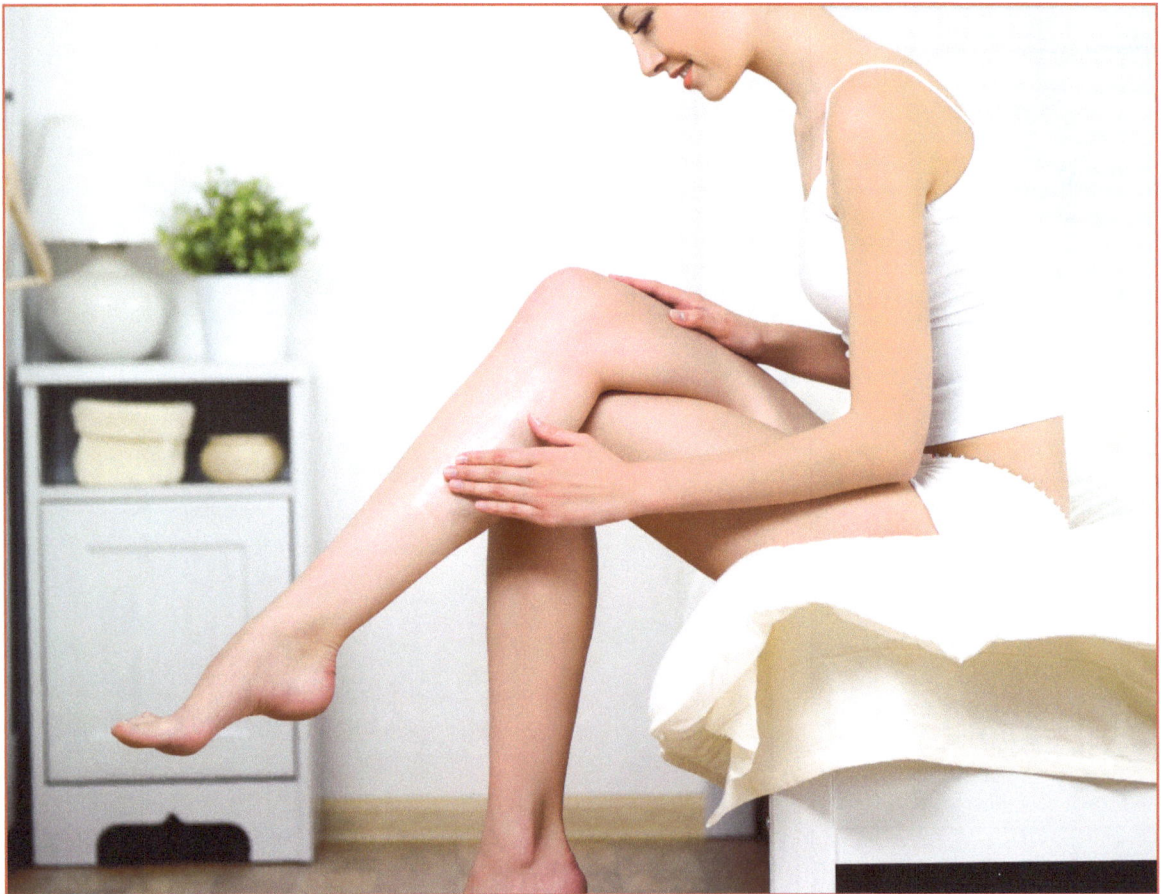

Chapter 7

My Lip Gloss is Pumping

Background: I would not want to take away from the classic red lipstick or the old Hollywood look. I love old Hollywood glamour, but if you don't choose the right shade of lipstick, it can make you look older. Who wants to look older? This is why the lip gloss is always a winner. It gives you the shine without making you look older. It also makes you look youthful and sexy with pouty lips.

With lip glosses, you don't have to worry about lip liners to frame your lips. Just glide it on, and you're ready to go. If you wear the lip gloss by itself, you will still achieve a young, fresh look all the time. There's nothing as sexy as a hot, full, high-shine lips.

Beauty Secrets:
1. **Basics: To achieve sexy lips, you need to start from the basics of keeping your lips moistened. Start by using the simple <u>lip balm</u> twice a day every day to keep your lips in its best condition.**
2. **The key secret is to use mostly <u>soft color lip gloss</u> like the nudes, the pinks, or just a clear color. However, darker shades are not completely ruled out because what is mostly important is that you're using lip gloss and not lipstick. Also, remember before you go to bed use lip balm or Vaseline to <u>keep your lips moistened throughout the night</u>. At night is the best time to really get your skin to hydrate.**

Sometimes, the lip glosses come in different flavors such as vanilla, cherry, and strawberry. It doesn't matter what flavor. This is only a matter of preference.

3. Avoid bad behaviors such as smoking cigarettes, chewing tobacco, or other substance abuse drugs. A set of dry lips can be easily moistened and youthful again, but a set of black lips can be challenging to reverse its color. So try to stop these bad behaviors. While you work on your behavior, you can still benefit from the look that a high-shine lip gloss offers. The effortless application is by using the applicator that it comes with and swiping the product onto your lips.

4. Imagine now with whitened set of teeth and high-shine glossy lips. If you follow these steps, you'll achieve sexy, voluptuous, shiny lips that would be attractive and noticeable.

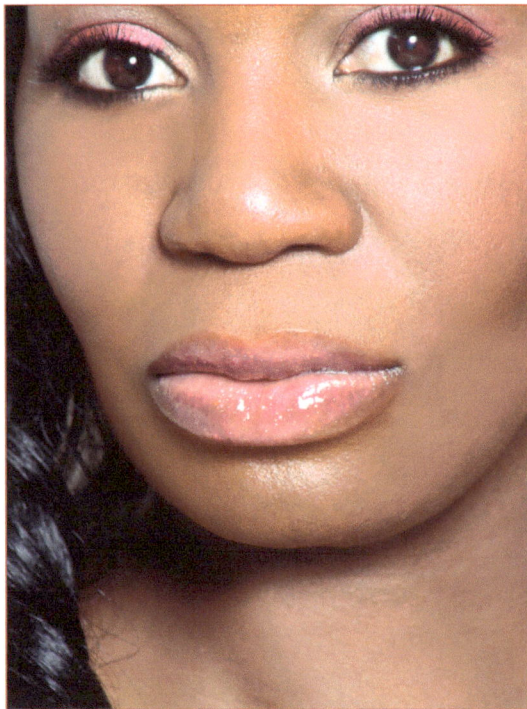

Beauty Beyond

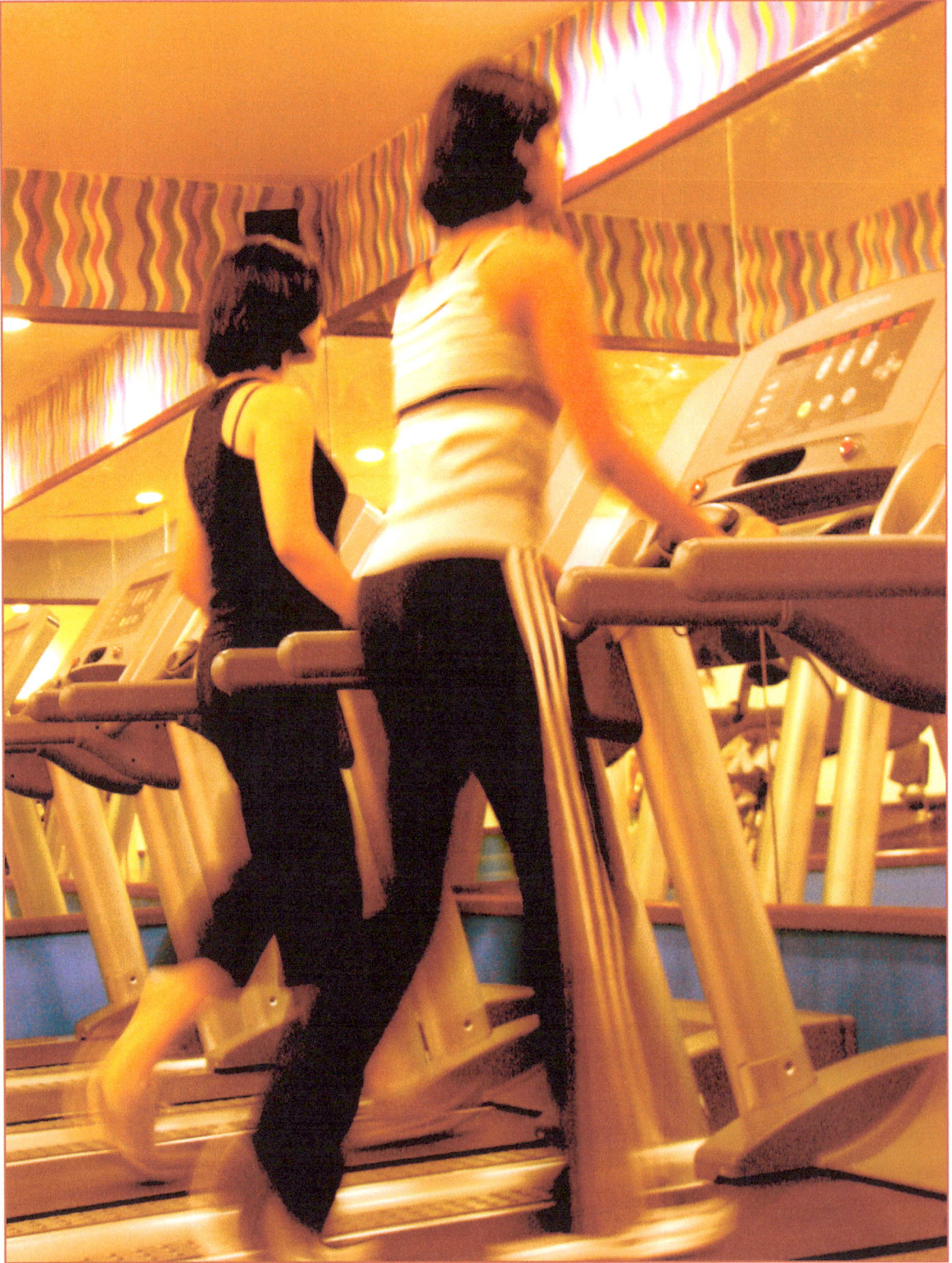

Chapter 8

Exercise: Sweat Time

Background: Weight loss is important to achieving youthful appearance. If you're a little overweight or obese and you want to look 10 years younger, the quicker way to attain this goal is to lose some weight. Being overweight makes you look older than you really are. It also causes other medical problems like high blood pressure, diabetes, blood clots etc. You will have to learn to commit to a reduced calorie diet and incorporate some healthy fruits and vegetables. You can adopt sample meals such as the following.

Breakfast @ 10AM: Have 2 slices of toast, an apple, and an 8-ounce glass of orange juice.

Snack @ 12PM: Have an 80-calories low-fat yoghurt with a bottle of water.

Lunch @ 2PM: You can do a chicken salad with low-fat dressing and a bottle of water.

Snack @ 4PM: Have a lunch snack with a fruit such as an orange, watermelon, or apple and a bottle of water.

Dinner @ 6PM: A small portion of rice, a larger portion of vegetables such as broccoli, a generous portion of lean protein such as grilled fish or chicken, and a bottle of water.

Snack @ 8PM: You can have a fruit again or a low-fat desert, and a cup of tea or a bottle of water.

You really don't want to eat more than 3 main meals of more than 2,000 calories and 2-3 snacks per day. Your goal should be to eat 5-6 small meals per day. You want to drink at least a bottle of water each time you eat something. You should be drinking a minimum of at least 8 glasses of 8-ounces of water per day. The more water you drink, the more you flush down the food for easy digestion and you're on your way to losing more weight. Also, don't forget that constipation can slow your metabolism which can delay you from achieving your weight loss. Therefore, drinking water, eating fibers, and eating fruits and vegetables will help you to have good bowel movements. So that leads me to inform you that bowel movements every day is important for smooth digestive processes. After all, it helps you to lose weight easily. If you ask me to tell you my personal weight loss secrets, they are: eating smaller portions, drinking lots of water, and moving my bowel daily. Once I'm able to do all three, I'm losing and maintaining my goal weight on a daily basis.

Keep your diet in check, and you can have a successful weight loss goal. You can't achieve your goal faster if your diet is bad and you're putting a lot of effort into exercising and vice versa. You have to put equal effort into both.

Your exercise plan should consist of some cardio, toning, stretching, and relaxation techniques. You can start with running on the tread mill or kickboxing for 30 minutes, and then you should consider yoga or pilates for 15 minutes at a time. Even if you can't do 30-60 minutes of workout at the same time, you can break it into two workouts per day. It's not about doing one long workout; it's about doing accumulated sets of workout for the time required. Before you start any exercise program, consult with your physician first.

Stress should be reduced in your daily lives as much as you can. By doing this alone would take away some wrinkle off your face. Adopt some relaxation techniques to keep you freshened at all times. Either yoga or pilates can help you to relax. Relaxation is needed to avoid aging appearances. You can also incorporate some meditation in the morning or before going to bed. Remember, your state of mind is important to help you inside and out.

Beauty Secrets:

1. Basics: Do some exercises <u>at least every other day</u> to achieve the best results. Your ideal goal should be 3 to 5 times per week.

2. The key secret is to do what you can. You have to be <u>persistent and consistent</u>. If you have to do <u>three sets of 10 minutes workout</u> at different times per day, then that is just as effective as doing <u>one 30 minutes workout</u>.

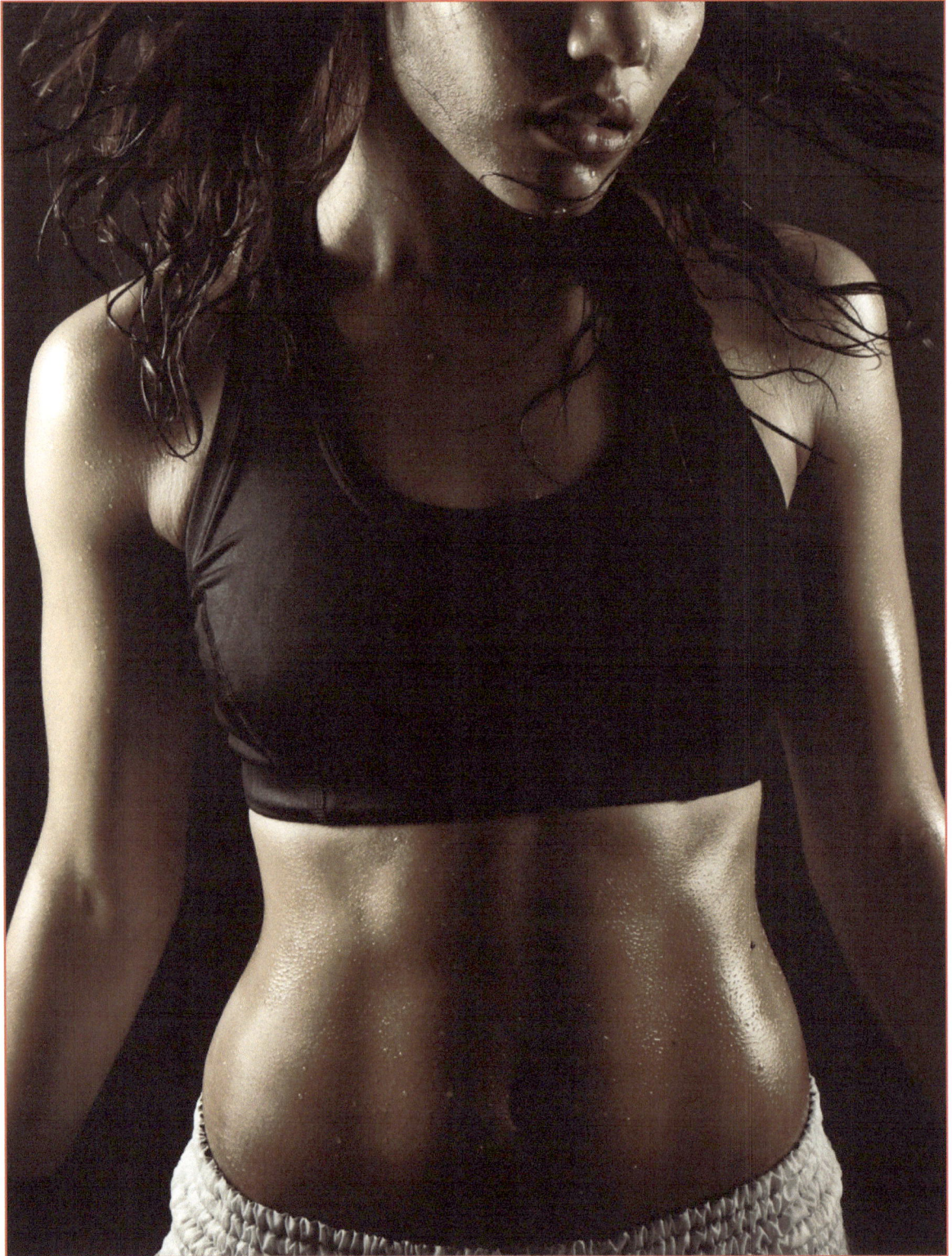

Chapter 9

Pre-Party GLOW

Background: I thought I should share with you one of my biggest beauty secrets. I found that each time after exercising I have an indescribable glow. When I workout during the weekend, I usually do it before doing my chores. After taking a shower, I noticed the same glow. So I said to myself that this glow must be something I need to have with me whenever I'm going out to an event. The glow is a rich, golden one that comes from within. It makes you look like you've been doing everything you're supposed to do such as eating your fruits and vegetables, drinking tons of water, and being stress free.

Beauty Secrets:
1. **Basics: Follow your basic workout plan as described in the previous chapter. If you're persistent and consistent, you wouldn't have a problem working out right before going out to an event.**
2. **The key secret is to workout within an hour of going out. If you workout several hours before, the extra glow wouldn't be as spectacular as within an hour. Upon working out and taking a shower, your skin glows. Your body's natural oils resurface which gives you the amazing glow that is enhanced with your lotion, dispersed and caressed across your body. Going out in the night, you'll be surprised with the many compliments you'll receive. Only you'll be able to know what your secret is and you'll be hooked.**

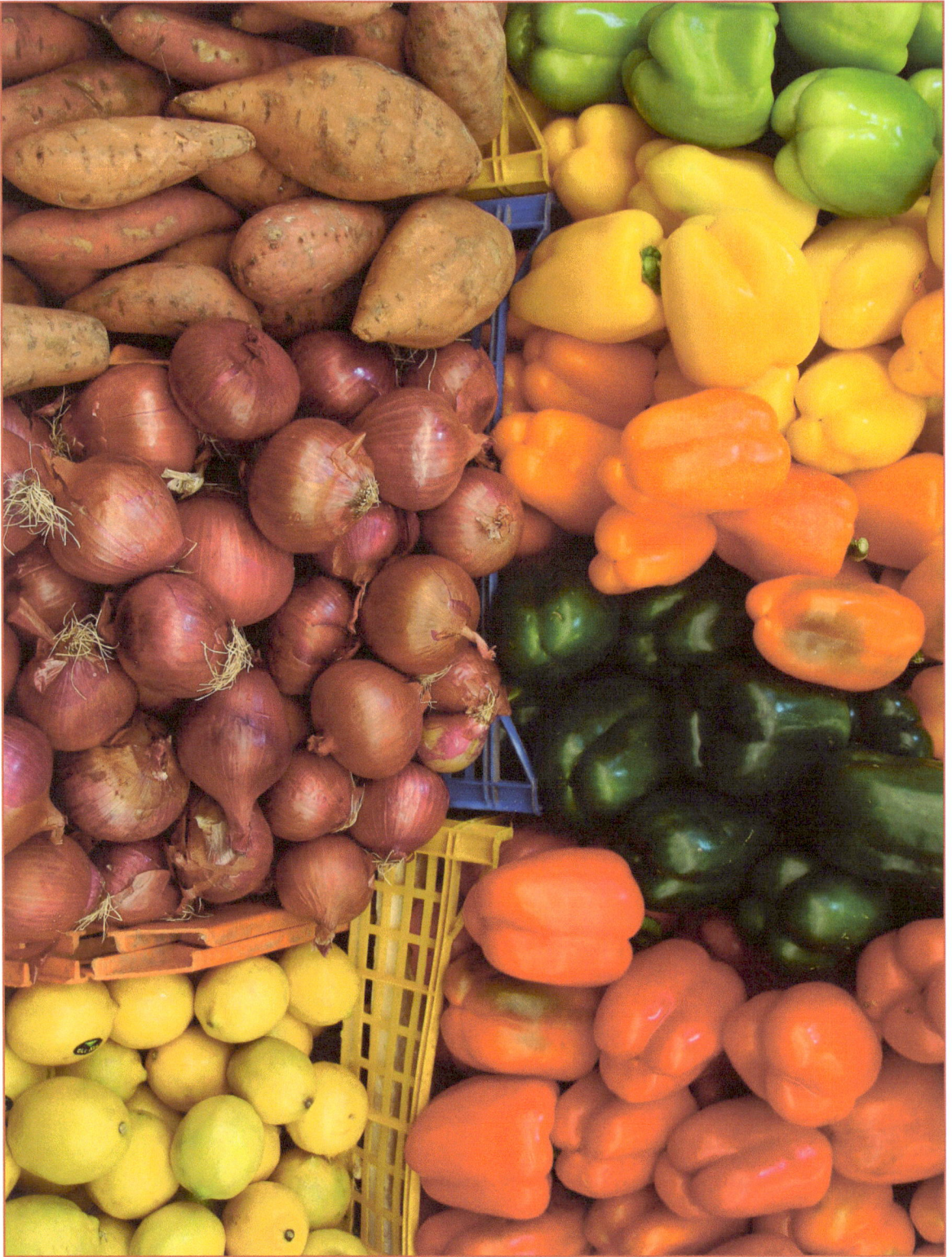

Chapter 10

Healthy Vitamins, Fruits, & Vegetables

Background: The secret to looking 10 years younger does not only apply to your outermost appearance. It's also about what you put inside. After discussing about healthy meals in the previous chapter, it's also important to incorporate daily vitamins, fruits and vegetables into your diet. Your body is a whole system, and it's impossible to eat enough fruits and vegetables per day even if you tried. So you can take your daily vitamins every day. Certain brands have higher amount of vegetables per serving.

Beauty Secrets:

1. **Basics: If you follow my sample meal with the workout plan in Chapter 8, you already know that you should be eating <u>at least 2-3 fruits per day</u>.**

2. **The key secret is that 2-3 fruits per day are really not enough. Therefore, <u>multivitamins</u> are good supplements to fruits and vegetables.**

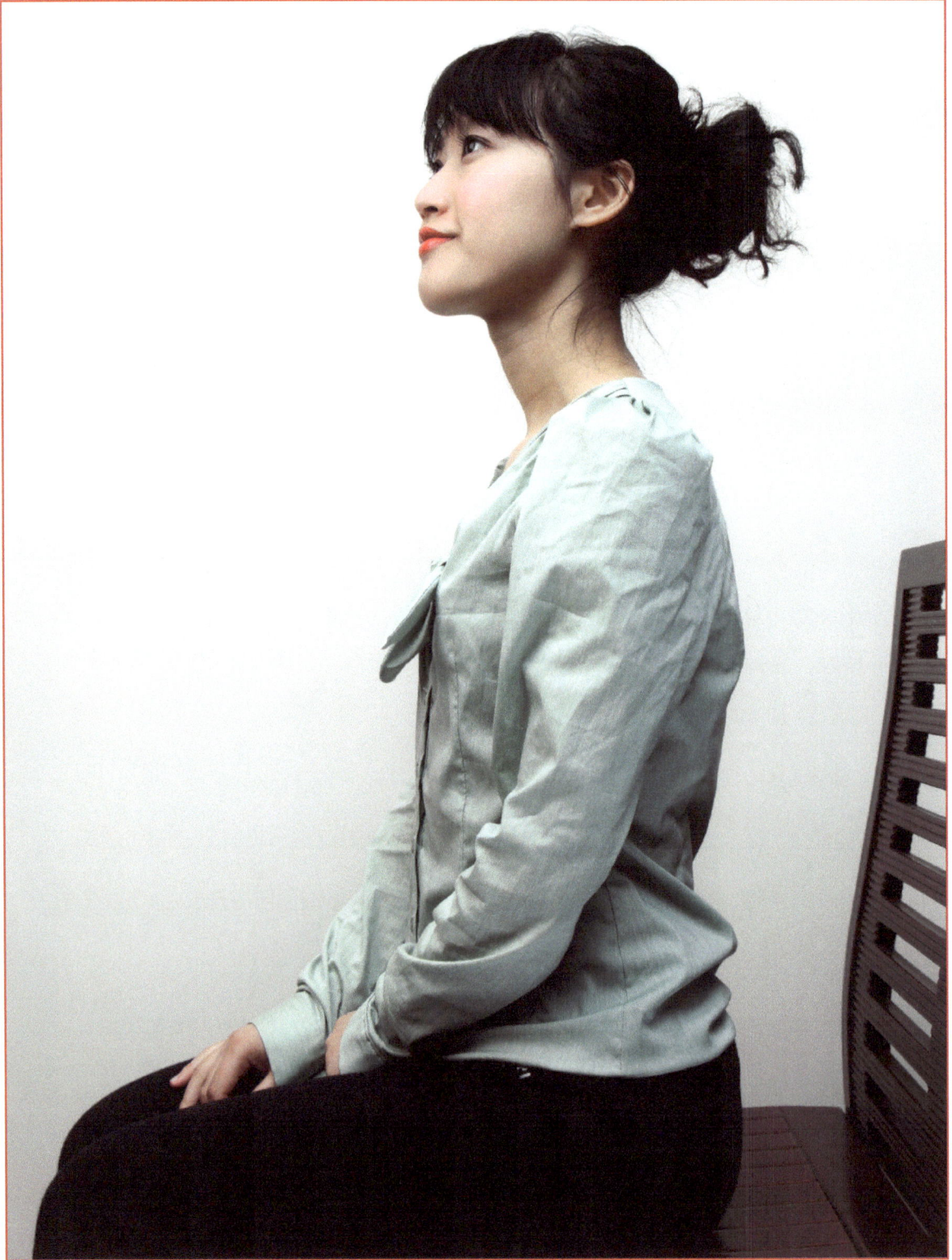

Chapter 11

Sit Like a Lady Please

Background: I've always wondered why some of us age just by the way we sit or carry ourselves. I've come to realize the importance in the way we keep our posture over the years. This is one of the reason why older people have osteoporosis or osteopenia which are loss of bone density depending on the severity. Either the way you sit or carry yourself is not the number one cause of osteoporosis or osteopenia. If you continuously sit or stand with a hunch back all day long, you're most likely to have bad posture. It's never too late to reverse that behavior if it hasn't already caused you a disfigured back.

There's a reason why models sit with their backs straight and they walk with their chests out. They do this because it's youthful to sit-up straight and walk with chest out while leaning backwards. I know it's easy to get carried away with other things going on around you than worry about the way you sit or walk. But all you can do is try and pay attention. It's just like anything else you do on a daily basis. If you put your mind to it, you'll see that sitting up straight will make you present yourself like a lady.

Beauty Secrets:

1. **Basics: Avoid habits such as sitting or walking with a hunch back.**

2. **The key secret is to <u>think tall</u> when you sit. When you <u>sit tall</u>, you look sexy, like a lady, and a lot younger.**

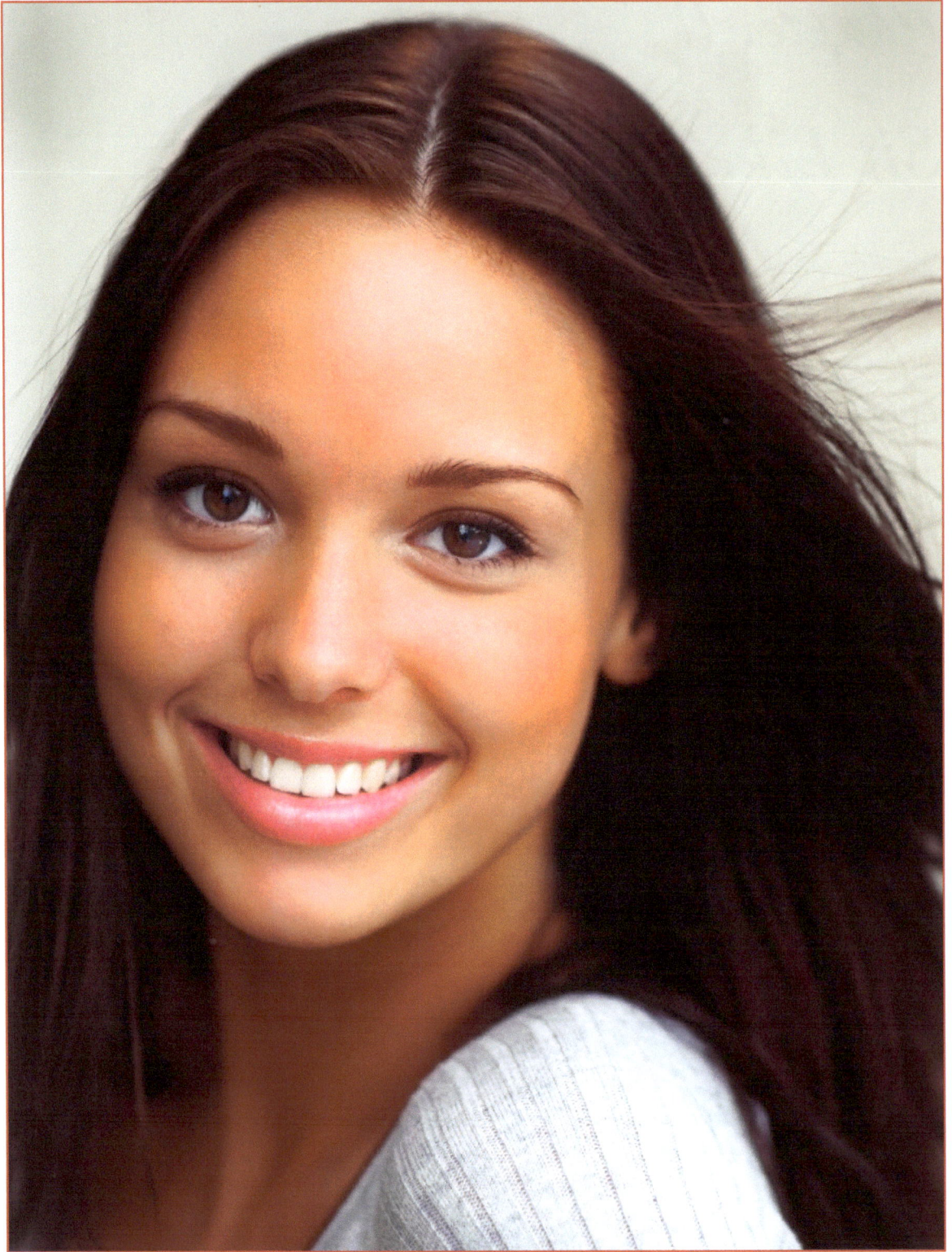

Chapter 12

Smiles—Say Cheese!

Background: I want to take this chapter to emphasize the beauty in smiling. There are so many things that go on in our lives on a daily basis. Some of them cause a lot of stress to the point where it transfers on to our personal lives. Anger can be as a result of the stress. Remember, it takes more facial muscles to frown than it is to smile. The more facial muscles you're using to frown, the more wrinkles you're most likely to have. So why put your facial muscles through all that stress and your face through all those wrinkles? Just smile!

Beauty Secrets:

1. **Basics: Follow the basics of having a <u>healthy set of teeth</u>.**

2. **The key secret is to realize that a smiley face indirectly brings out the youth in you, but a <u>smiley face with healthy whitened teeth</u>, and high-shined lip gloss, takes it to a whole new level of youthfulness.**

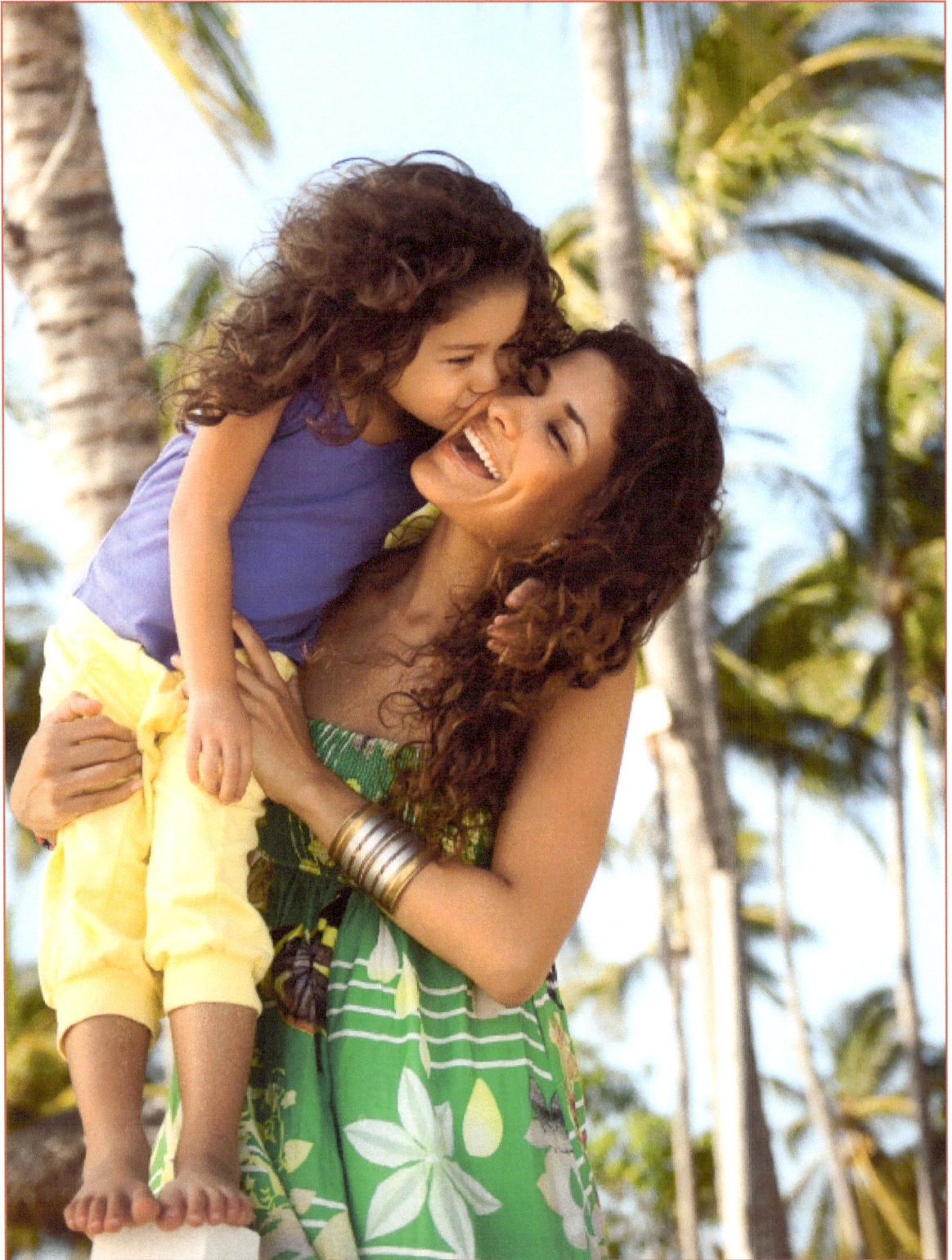

Chapter 13

Bring Out the Child in You

Background: I usually think that there's nothing as free-spirited as acting as a child once in a while. I also think sometimes we spend so much time being too serious and taking ourselves too seriously that we forget to relax, be playful, and have fun. Kids are kids because they act like kids and have fun. They have nothing to worry about, and they just have a good time. Sometimes, we need to do this once in a while. This is why it's okay to come out of your comfort zone and play with your children if you have some. They keep you young and on your toes. You may even get some exercises while you're at it. If you don't have any children, you can still find ways to be playful some times.

Beauty Secrets:

1. **Basics: To be a child at heart, you have to <u>be yourself</u>.**

2. **The key secret to being a child at heart is to <u>learn to relax</u>, <u>be playful</u> and <u>don't take yourself too seriously</u>.**

Chapter 14

Laughter is Youthful

Background: Just like many beauty secrets of anti-aging, good laughter can help you to look 10 years younger. Laughter is a good medicine. Laughter is important because it relaxes you, and if you're relaxed most of the time, you skin is farther away from aging. Sometimes aging is not only about the skin, but it's about the way you feel. If you're always unhappy, it will translate in the way you look and can make you age faster.

Beauty Secrets:

1. Basics: Again, <u>be yourself</u> and don't be up-tight.

2. The key secret to making laughter an anti-aging recommendation is to have a <u>great sense of humor</u>. Have a <u>good outlook in life</u>.

3. Every now and then, go to a <u>comedy show</u>. You'll have a good laugh. It's <u>therapeutic</u>. You'll be surprised to see how much stress is released and how good you'll feel afterwards.

Chapter 15

Positivity is Anti-Aging

Background: If you're thinking about achieving youthful appearance, you have to be a positive person. You have to surround yourself with positive people. Positivity takes you far in life. If you're positive, your conscience can be clear, you can have a feel-good personality, and your skin is free of stress reactants. Stress can activate the process of inflammation in our body and chronically contribute to aging process. Sometimes, stress can cause other medical problems such as ulcers and high blood pressure. These are serious problems that can be prevented. So, staying healthy and being positive are important to reducing inflammation, staying young, and vibrant. Like someone previously said "Wellness is the absence of inflammation."

Beauty Secrets:

1. **Basics: A positive minded person could mean <u>longevity</u>. As they say, if you do well, you may live longer. Is this true though?**

2. **The key secret to looking 10 years younger is to <u>be positive</u>, <u>think positive</u>, and <u>do positive things</u>.**

3. **It is therapeutic to be positive, and it <u>will show on your skin</u>.**

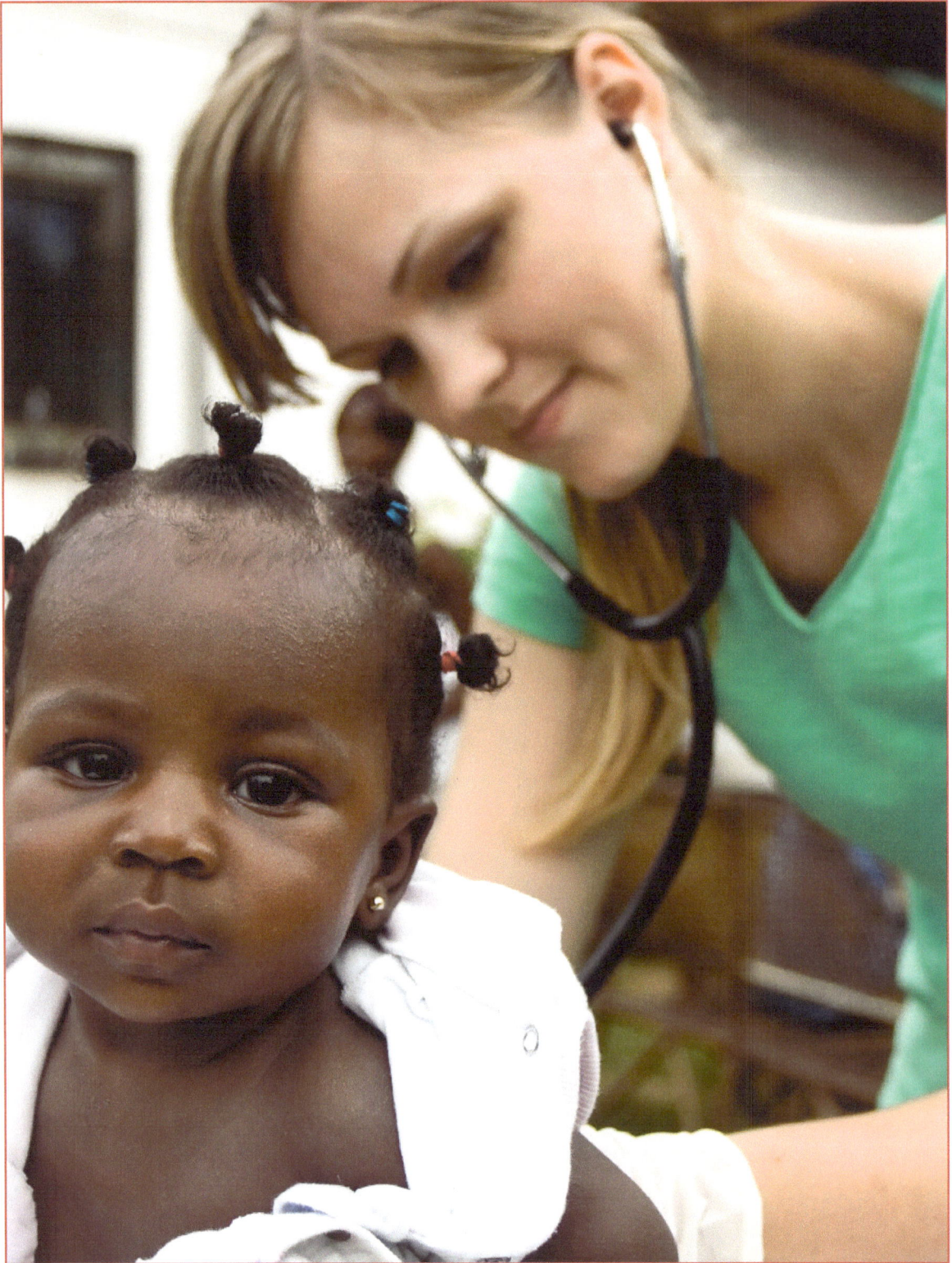

Chapter 16

Eternity LOVE

Background: It is important to understand who you are, what you do, and how what you do can affect your way of life. If your way of live is negative or does not bring out love, happiness, and positivity, it shows on your outer appearance. This is because your skin gets beat up and takes the suffering. Therefore, show some love and receive some love. Love is the greatest gift in life.

Beauty Secrets:

1. **Basics:** <u>**Surround yourself**</u> **with love.**

2. **The key secret to how love can help you look 10 years younger is to** <u>first love yourself</u>. **Give love to others, and you'll receive love. Don't worry about receiving; just give instead. When you continue to give love, you'll receive some day. When you're all about love, the goodness in the interior will spill to the exterior. This attitude of love will bring a glow from within that helps to keep a youthful appearance.**

Conclusion

I hope with this book you've been able to discover my *white* beauty secrets to looking 10 years younger and more. Let's face it; there are many anti-aging products out there to use to prevent wrinkles, decrease pores and puffy eyes. But they are expensive, and they probably require doing invasive procedures. Besides, there aren't any magic pills, creams, ointments, or serums. However, there are things you can do to enhance your facial features and your inner beauty that brings out your natural beauty and helps you to look 10 years younger. This is what sets this book apart. It helps you to achieve youthful appearance with unique and inexpensive beauty regime.

By following my *white* beauty regime, you'll see the importance of keeping certain parts of your body in its whitest color. The whiter your eyes, the sexier they are. The whiter your teeth are, the brighter your smile. The clearer your nails are, the healthier they look. They all have one thing in common and that is –youthfulness. Trust me; if you keep everything white, or at least think of the importance of white in anti-aging, you're doing great. Now go out there, be fabulous and use these secrets to look 10 years younger and vibrant like you deserve.